M000285343

ISBN: 978-0-692-92392-4 (softcover)

ISBN: 978-0-692-92393-1 (eBook)

www.DementiaGuiltGuide.com

Dawna Cappello and Susan Heller

Contents

Foreword

To my readers; here is what I want you to know.

I wrote this short book because if you are reading it, you are likely in hell or witnessing it. I am going to be honest about the process that we went through and I am going to offer suggestions, alternatives, and options, so that you and your loved ones do not have to suffer as we did.

My way of sharing with you some of the tools I created along the way are marked with this sign: ⌘. In the world of Mac computers, that clover-leaf is designated the "Command" key, which is what I want to give you for reasons that will become clear as you move through this narrative. Command over what happens in terms of how you deal with it and what you *can* do about the bits you can't actually do anything about.

The three of us; my husband Michael, his mother, (I call her Mom) and I, each had our own reasons for being 100% loyal to our promise to keep my father-in-law at home and to never send him away to a residential nursing facility.

As you read this book, you will likely realize that we were all in denial, but we had made a promise to Lou and to one another, not to betray him. In hindsight, we were 100% wrong about the decisions we made. But we were doing the best we could with the information we had at the time.

Here is the information we now know.
My heartfelt wish is that it helps you and yours.

Dawna Cappello

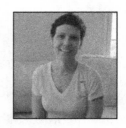

I spent almost a decade taking care of my father-in-law who was suffering from multiple causes of dementia. Taking on the additional role of family spokesperson meant I was providing physical, emotional, psychological, social, and economic guidance. I truly understand the depth of the drama, the fear, and the frustration.

I don't want anybody to go through what we went through. **MISFIRE** is my way of ensuring nobody has to.

I have degrees in business and psychology. I even worked as a crisis counselor, a recreational therapist and a cognitive trainer for an Alzheimer's Resource Center, but I wasn't prepared for what happened when dementia hit my family.

I'm passionate about helping others who are looking at the possibility of confronting the same issues or are currently living in a similar situation. Which is why I also became credentialed as a dementia specialist, and why this book came about.

I want you to know, you have choices.

For more information, or to schedule a Presentation on-site or by Skype, visit the Website: www.DementiaGuiltGuide.com

Susan Heller

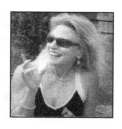

At nine years old, I was dissecting shark eyeballs that I kept in an olive jar in the refrigerator. How do you top that? My answer was to parlay my ability to turn things sideways or inside out for a unique view. I became a highly visual writer, producer, and director.

In terms of what I do, I guess eclectic describes it best. I author and co-author; biographies, stories, and novels. I also write a wide range of articles from occasional rants about the exigencies of life, to PR pieces and book reviews. Creating Business Development Communications and Marketing Tools for an international Ports Stevedoring company was fun. Creating an entire Show Bible for an upcoming episodic TV series was even funner (she said, invoking a writer's privilege to mess with language). Writing, producing, and directing a private teaser (called "FIRESTORM") for investors of a TV series was a blast.

Working with professionals is my absolute favorite thing to do. And by "professionals" I mean anybody, at any level, in or outside of any profession, who takes their project and creativity seriously enough to enjoy the process and treat everyone along the way with consideration and respect. That, to me, is the *funnest* thing of all.

Dawna Cappello is someone I know professionally and personally. As soon as I read her journal, I knew I wanted to help create a compelling and succinct narrative that could help preclude the suffering of others.

For more information, or to see additional samples of Susan's work, visit the Website: www.DementiaGuiltGuide.com

Dawna Cappello and Susan Heller

Introduction

ROBIN WILLIAMS
August 11, 2014

** Robin Williams Died.

** The Mass Media went berserk.

** The world lost a heroic man and a genius.

** As a world-wide celebrity, he had access to the best doctors and medical care.

** Robin's wife, Susan Schneider Williams, undertook a journey to find a way to educate the medical community about Lewy Body Dementia.

LOUIS CAPPELLO
April 21, 2016

** Lou Cappello Died.

** The Mass Media was silent.

** The world lost an extraordinary father and husband.

** As a working-class man, he had access to doctors and medical care.

** Lou's daughter-in-law, Dawna Cappello, undertook a journey to preclude other families from going through what hers did with Lewy Body Dementia.

Lou Cappello died in April 2016, and this story is being written in 2017, so you may have heard the term *Lewy Body Dementia* because of the suicide of Robin Williams. It wasn't until I was working on this book with Susan Heller that we came across an article by his wife, Susan Schneider Williams, written for the Official Journal of the American Academy of Neurology, in September 2016. **

What happened to Robin Williams is exactly what happened to my father-in-law Lou, though the process was mirrored back-to-front. Lou's descent began with Parkinson's disease and ended with Lewy Body Dementia; Robin's nightmare apparently began (though no one knew it at the time) with Lewy Body Dementia and ended with Parkinson's disease.

Susan Schneider Williams' article is an outreach directed toward the medical profession. This book is the working man's version of that outreach, directed to the family and friends of those dealing with these complex and difficult diseases.

*   *   *

Chapter 1
OMG! Are You Kidding Me?

My view of the road became distorted and turned into a kind of hazy tunnel vision. The tree line whipping by me on both sides looked like green paint splattered haphazardly on a blank canvas. Tears were rolling down my cheeks and literally forming puddles in my lap. I started yelling. *"WHY?! Why is this happening?"*

Months and months of sleepless nights, it was relentless. My husband, my mother-in-law, and I, getting up every night, over and over and over; we were beyond exhausted. We were frightened, frustrated, and at our wits end. My father-in-law Lou, had Parkinson's disease which is challenging to begin with, but things were going from bad to much worse. It looked like he had dementia too. Come to find out, that is not uncommon among victims of Parkinson's disease.

Lou was hearing voices and seeing people who were coming to get him, he was terribly frightened. At the time, we thought they were delusions and we believed our constant and repeated reassurances that nobody was there and that everything was okay would relieve his anxiety and paranoia. But unbeknownst to us, from his perspective, he was telling the God's honest truth. His brain was delivering information to his eyes and ears that was as real to him as the seat that you're sitting on is to you. So Lou was reacting the way any of us would if we were being menaced and our lives were being threatened. My mother-in-law Barbara and my husband Michael were horrified that Lou thought anyone wanted to do him harm.

*   *   *

I believe in personal accountability. I also believe each one of us is here to do what we can, as Dr. Michael

Beckwith artfully puts it, "…to be a beneficial presence on the planet." Participating in this Earth-walk can be both a brutal and exhilarating experience. So my intent is to look for the positive and share what I have learned about the dark side. Because we are all on the same journey; that of being a self-aware somebody in space and time.

That said, I didn't feel like I was on the planet, I felt like I was in hell and I was howling my fear and fury at the heavens. When comedians talk about the ugly-cry they often get a laugh, but that is exactly what I was doing; sobbing, hyperventilating, screaming myself hoarse.

Eyes closed, I told myself to snap out of it and to just deal with it. I kept trying to calm down and then something very strange happened. Just like that, I became completely still. Four words, one at a time, dropped into my head. "You. Have. No. Control."

Okay, did I just hear from God, or am I doing my own version of Lou, hearing things? But I knew I wasn't making it up. Nothing like that had ever happened to me before. And it was true. I could not begin to control what was going on in Lou's head, in his heart, and his body…what a relief.

Suddenly, I was back to furious.

Eyes turned skyward, I screamed like a banshee, *"Are you freaking kidding me? Again?! WTF?"* How many times was I going to have to relearn the fact that I have no control over anything? *"I KNOW I don't have control. THANK YOU very much! REALLY?"*

My heart was racing, practically beating out of my chest, and I may have hammered the steering wheel with my open palms four hundred times. Finally, I snapped back into time and the see-saw shifted again.

I sat without moving, without speaking; barely breathing. I'd been driving for close to twenty minutes without ever once looking at the road. How the hell did I get home? I knew I was exhausted, oh my God, did I fall asleep at the wheel? I don't remember steering, I don't remember putting on my blinker, I don't remember turning off of the highway. I wasn't driving, but somehow I arrived safely. Then it hit me. Now my tears were soft and in deep gratitude, and this time when I gazed skyward all I could say was, *"Thank you."*

I sat quietly allowing my physiology to catch up with the peace that was filling my soul and the next thing I heard was, "Share your story; help others." And this time there was absolutely no doubt in my mind. We were witnessing the trauma of Parkinson's disease and the drama of dementia, and Somebody was telling me that I needed to tell others, so they wouldn't make all the same mistakes we did.

It was time to sit down and write.

*   *   *

Chapter 2
Lou Who?

My father-in-law was one of the lucky ones. He was second generation Italian and had a great childhood. His father came over from Italy circa 1930, and Lou was born in New Haven, Connecticut. Like many children of first generation immigrants, Lou was a hard worker who, at age seventeen, began working at a bakery and soon made enough money to buy a small boat - his favorite place in the world to spend his free time.

He was soft spoken, a man of few words, and was most comfortable when he was in his own company. He didn't even notice that there was a girl who lived just across the street from the marina who watched him coming and going. That shy sixteen-year-old was my mother-in-law, Barbara. In 1958, Barbara talked a friend into coming with her, they walked over to Lou while he was working on his boat and struck up a conversation. Lou and Barbara began dating.

Lou's upbringing instilled in him a deep connection with family, a strong work ethic, and a clear understanding of what it meant to be considered a man of integrity. He was funny, he was handsome, with a very contagious smile. Barbara was still shy and didn't talk much about herself or her family. It was two full years before Lou learned why she was reluctant to talk, and how truly dark her childhood had been. She had been sexually abused and spent her young life living in an orphanage or at the homes of various family members. Finally, one week after her 21st birthday, on October 1st, 1963, Lou was able to keep the promise he had made to himself. He married Barbara and they moved out of town.

For six years Lou worked at the bakery, then his culture and his protective sensibilities for his wife led him to apply to a communications company where he could be in a stable full-time job with benefits. Time to start a family.

If Lou was lucky, Barbara was blessed. Despite the trauma of her early years, she had an incredible disposition. She was kind, good natured, and gave unconditionally to everyone in her life. No one, no church, no institution had to teach her that, it's just who she was. The fact that Lou had rescued her from her fractured home meant she was bound to him, both by love and gratitude. It was Barbara who took care of Lou's mother when she became ill and moved into their family home.

They were a sweet couple. Barbara stood 5'6" and had a lovely figure. Lou was 5'8", with a strong build, and was particularly proud of his thick, wavy, Italian hair. Married for almost fifty-three years, they had lived forty-seven of them in the same home. Everyone; friends, family members, as well as any unattached animal was welcome, anytime.

*　　　　*　　　　*

Chapter 3
My Guy

So, remember the see-saw metaphor from Chapter 1? If, for any reason, you put the book down, let me quickly revisit it; up, down, up, down, up, down; pretty much the definition of most people's lives.

The reason I can write this, is that I, like Lou, am one of the lucky ones. And I know it. Lou's son Michael is what I would call an elegant soul, an ethical man, and a guy with a boundless heart. Just so you know, I'm not gushing. We've been together for twelve years and the guy has seen me through some ridiculously awful times. I trust him with my life.

Michael has an unusual quality, one you don't find that often in a man – he is an empath. If you're not familiar with the word, it means that someone is so deeply connected to another, they literally experience the emotions and consequences, both beneficial and deleterious, of their loved one. In some ways, you might call it a parallel reality.

When Michael was twenty-seven years old, his very best friend was dying of cancer. Chemotherapy meant losing her hair. Simultaneously, Michael began to lose his hair as well; it was falling out in clumps every time he showered.

Medically, alopecia is considered an autoimmune disease; however, I think that the timing pretty much says it. And when you read about what Michael did when the world turned upside-down for Lou; how he stepped up and stepped in, in a thousand different ways, for everyone involved, you'll come to understand why I consider him something of a hero and a superior role-model.

Michael's best friend died, and he still has alopecia, but the man knows who he is, so the loss of his hair no longer matters.

*   *   *

Chapter 4
Pronounced: /'daʊn/a

Right about now you've got to be wondering who I am. Some of the labels that would make sense to you are; Type-A personality, highly energetic (on occasion to the point of hyper), very organized (so much so that even my vacuum lines in the carpet have to be straight), and someone who sees every new skill, profession, or vocation as a total challenge. I want to be good at it. No wait, I want to be great.

"So what," you say, "I know lots of people like that," however, most Type-A personalities are not goodie-two-shoes, and trust me, I am. I can be tough as nails, I'm tenacious as hell, and probably could have been a good drill sergeant, except for the fact that I don't much appreciate authority. And here is the addendum to the goodie-two-shoes comment; unlike a good drill sergeant, I am hyperconscious of other people's feelings and don't want anyone to be ashamed, upset, or scared. Ever. I have a smile three-yards-wide, and when I'm not screaming skyward, I'm usually laughing, singing, or dancing.

Full disclosure, I'm not soft-spoken as much as I am out-spoken. I have a tinge of a whiskey voice, which trust me, gets heard above the cacophony of normal female chatter. Some, or maybe all, of the above personality traits can be traced to the fact that I have been on my own since I was sixteen-years-old.

Together for twelve years, married for eight, Michael and I had actually been in each other's orbit, in school and as friends, for over thirty-three years. Which is why we knew when we were married in 2009, we had to have a friend standing at my father-in-law's side because the drama was already in progress.

Michael would have no one but his father as his best man at our wedding. However, because of the progression of Lou's Parkinson's disease, which had been diagnosed thirteen years earlier, we knew he could not stand on his own without assistance when it was time to make the toast. But we could not let Lou know that we knew. It all had to appear very natural and spontaneous.

Have I mentioned the word stubborn? Also known as: adamant, inflexible, intractable, or just plain bull-headed. You could pretty much apply any of those adjectives to Lou, to Michael, and once again, full disclosure, to me as well. On the other hand, although I can out-stubborn a cat, when it comes to being flexible about what needs to happen to keep the people I love safe, I will bend like a reed in the wind.

For Lou, that stubborn personality trait stood him in good stead as a business manager, an entrepreneur, and as a man determined to give his family the best life possible. However, when he got sick, it turned on him in the worst way possible.

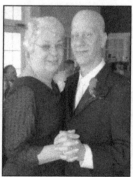 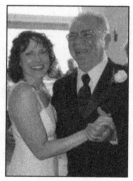

The picture of me with my father-in-law is one of the reasons Michael and I believe in miracles. The wedding photographer caught the only time Lou smiled in seven years.

*　　　　*　　　　*

Chapter 5
Standing By...

Mom had always been proud of the fact that she was a great cook. Everybody said so, especially Lou. So we were all stunned when he started to refuse to eat anything she made him. And I mean *anything*. If she was the one who poured frosted flakes into a bowl, they were inedible. Mom tried everything. She offered him multiple options, then made special shopping trips to get him what he said he wanted. To no avail. His stomach hurt, he was experiencing constipation, and he was convinced it was because Mom had done something to the food.

Apparently, Robin Williams also experienced digestion issues, but because the symptoms would come and go, they were considered repercussions of fear and anxiety. OMG! That was the very same information we were given by our doctors. It's so very frustrating because since the 1980's, it has been well known that taste and smell impairment are classic symptoms of Parkinson's disease *and* Lewy Body Dementia. If we had known that, it could have alleviated the additional guilt, upset, and stress that was piling up on us for not being able to give Lou what he needed.

Instead, we did the same things for Lou that Susan did for Robin; we had him tested. From blood-work to a colonoscopy to an endoscopy; none of them came back abnormal. Was Lou simply becoming a hypochondriac?

*   *   *

I'm getting a little ahead of myself, but I thought it important that you understand the characters and the context involved, including the fact that Michael and I were living together in an apartment when we realized Lou and Mom were having incredible trouble dealing with the reality of his Parkinson's disease. The symptoms are tough, and not every person will experience all of them; they include tremors and shaking, loss of smell, trouble sleeping, a stiff body and shuffling of feet while walking, constipation, a constant blank stare, a hunched body position, and hallucinations; a symptom we didn't know about and did not understand.

So Mom, Michael, and I had a conversation and agreed that the best way Michael and I could step-up our ability to help Lou, was for us to move into a house they owned that was only two doors away from where they lived. The year was 2007.

There wasn't any question about making the move. Standing by each other was something the Cappello's did well. My amazing husband stood by me during a horrific and very nearly fatal bout of appendicitis and for the years it took me to recover afterwards. Mom is the mother I never had. She loved me, she treated me as her own, and stronger by far than any blood connection, I was her daughter. Lou was kind and funny, a salt-of-the-earth type of guy who totally accepted me for me. I finally had the family I had longed for so desperately, perhaps one of the greatest gifts anyone could ever receive. There was no way I was going to let them down.

I'm going to repeat something I said in the Foreword; if you are reading this, you are likely in a living hell. Please understand there is hope, there is love, and there is peace. Sharing how crazy and dark things can get and then showing how there can still be laughter and times of grace, including deepening the connections with other caregivers, is what will ultimately get you through, as it did the three of us.

*   *   *

Chapter 6
The De-Construction

This might be when I started to wonder just who was in control of my life. And as it happens, that corny (often utterly infuriating) saying--things always work out for the best--was already operating behind the scenes. In short, here's how the next five years played out:

- I spent time volunteering at the Alzheimer's Resource Center of Connecticut residential facility, and received invaluable training and hands-on experience.
- I was *not* accepted into the graduate program that I'd applied for. (Wait a minute, wait a minute! I graduated summa-cum-laude, got an "A" on my final psych project, and had incredible references…what the heck was going on and what the heck was I going to do instead?)
- I was then hired as a Recreational Therapist at the Alzheimer's Resource Center.

By this time, even though we lived only two houses away, Michael and I found ourselves practically living with Lou and Mom (which answers the question of what I was going to be doing with all my "free" time). Lou was falling a lot, he was having all kinds of issues, the Parkinson's was getting much worse.

One night, at three in the morning, Mom called us in a complete panic; Lou had fallen and smashed his head. There was no time to dress, we actually streaked across the cul-de-sac. Michael and I were there almost before she hung up the phone.

That was when we decided the only way this was going to work for Lou and Mom, and prevent the neighbors from having to call the police on us for indecent exposure, was to build an accessory apartment above their house. Maybe then Michael could actually get some sleep. As a technical expert with his company, he was on call 24/7/365, the all-nighters with Lou were especially hard on him.

So we decided to start construction right away and because I have a background in property development, it made sense for me to act as the general contractor on the job.

That was when the proverbial s*** really hit the fan. We had no idea the chaos of construction was going to trigger Lou in so many ways and things immediately ballooned out of control.

The Lewy Body Dementia (we later learned) was starting to take over his brain. From Lou's perspective, his house was being invaded. Every construction worker was the enemy. He was raging and confrontational, then he'd become silent and withdrawn. He knew that we were conspiring against him to force him out of his home so that we could take over.

Eventually, like a baby just learning to walk, Lou became physically very unstable. One of us had to follow behind him whenever he began to aimlessly wander. Before you ask, if you haven't already, why we couldn't just insist he stay in one place, or design some sort of protective custody in the house, it's important to remember (and you may already be up against the same issue) that regardless of what Michael, Mom, and I said and irrespective of the strategies we devised, the law of the land says that Lou was an adult man and had the right to do or not do anything he chose at any given moment.

At one point, Mom was behind him as he fumbled his way down the stairs into the basement. He stood there, slowly looking right and left, then he collapsed to the ground sobbing, his shoulders shaking. "They gave away all of my stuff, they gave away all of my stuff."

Like many basements (and after forty-seven years) the space had become a catch-all for the family detritus down through the decades. We did give some stuff away, but mostly we tossed out trash and made room so the construction workers could store their tools. We kept trying to explain; all of us crying, yelling, and talking at once. Lou couldn't hear a single word. His brain had turned off his ears.

*   *   *

Chapter 7
180° x 180°

Lou was a successful executive so when he was only forty-eight he was offered what's known in the corporate world as "a golden parachute". He jumped at the opportunity. Early retirement meant that he could start a home improvement and remodeling business with a close friend, something he'd always wanted to do.

As he was building his new business, Lou's mother was diagnosed with Alzheimer's disease. He and Mom did what the Cappello's always did; they took her into their home to care for her. Eventually, Grandma C., became so ill that they had to put her into a residential facility. The upset and guilt around that event was part of the reason Lou was afraid the same thing would happen to him, and another reason why Mom promised she would never, ever, do any such thing.

Running his own company meant Lou also had time to enjoy a very active lifestyle that included racquetball, hiking, fishing, and boating. Three years later, Lou was thrilled when he had the chance to buy a marina in Cape Cod at which point Lady Fate stepped in; his old company reached out and made him an offer he couldn't refuse. Lou went back to work.

One of the benefits of Lou's return to the corporate world was that he was finally able to entice Michael into applying for a job with his company. Michael was hired on his own merits but if you've learned anything about the personalities of the men in this story so far, you won't be surprised that he felt compelled to work three times harder than anyone else to prove he deserved the job.

Five years later Lou retired again, he had been diagnosed with Parkinson's disease at the age of fifty-five.

He sold the marina and became very proactive in terms of dealing with his diagnosis. He led the Parkinson's disease meetings in his area, he got himself into medication trials, and though he could no longer rocket around a racquetball court, he could and did play a mean game of Ping-Pong at the town senior center.

The other thing Lou did for himself at age sixty-two was buy his dream car. Something about the combination of his dark Italian hair blowing in the wind as he tooled about town in his bright red Mercedes made Lou feel like he was on top of the world.

* * *

Chapter 8
3.2 on the Richter Scale

Early morning sunlight streamed in the windows as I was buzzing around cleaning the apartment before heading out to work. I leaned over to push the vacuum's ON button, and found my knees buckling as the floor shook to the accompaniment of a tremendous crash. Earthquake? Lou!

At this time, Lou was still able to be on his own. I was the only one home that morning, but just in case, I had left the door to the connecting stairwell open. *"Hey Dad, is everything okay?"* He responded quickly but in a whisper, "No." It was our first year in the new apartment and I was still trying to figure out personal boundaries. I didn't want to humiliate him, nor did I want to catch an eye-full. I called out, *"Are you dressed?"* His voice stronger, he muttered, "Yes. Are you?"

Now laughing, I headed down the stairs to find him flat on his back in the hallway leading to the kitchen. *"Are you hurt?"* He shook his head. I bent down and eased him into a standing position, then carefully walked him to a chair. I asked again if he was hurt. The only words he could muster were, "Only my pride." The embarrassed look on his face had already told me that.

Lou was still able to make occasional trips to the casino with Mom, which kept him walking long distances (if you've never been in a Connecticut casino before, you need to know that the hallways go on for miles). To us, Lou appeared cognitively aware, so he was in charge of taking his medications. The thought never occurred to us to challenge that. But, the dementia was progressing.

On occasion, his random confusion would suddenly spill over into aggression in the form of verbal combat. Mom was having a very difficult time, nothing she said or did was right or pleased him and she--actually all three of us--were taking it personally. In hindsight, it's clear that the mood swings, the selfishness, the constant criticism; everything was due to the dual monsters invading his brain and his nervous system. And even after Lou was diagnosed with Lewy Body Dementia, nobody explained to us that that specific diagnosis entailed an entirely unique constellation of symptoms. So we didn't know that we didn't know.

Which is why I want you to know, when you're in the middle of it, and the family member or friend you're dealing with appears to be in their right mind a good part of the time, all you can do is manage the moment the best way you can. Even if we had understood what was going on, forcing Lou to do anything that didn't make sense to him or that he didn't want to do, engendered a massive battle.

No matter what we did or didn't do, no matter how we handled or didn't handle it, how we screamed, shouted, fought, doubted, loved, or hated, the stomach-churning upset rattled every physical and emotional bone in our bodies.

*   *   *

Chapter 9
Oh, Dear God. What Have We Done?

Michael and I had been wracking our brains for ways to shift Lou's focus to a positive place, but just as important was finding a way to alleviate the pressure for Mom. She had been taking care of Lou and covering for him with friends and family for more years than she let on. Her life was no longer the same; her loving husband had turned into an angry and dissatisfied bully. She felt like a slave and was crying every day. In despair, she admitted to me that she was afraid she was going to die before Lou did, from a stroke or a heart attack.

It was 2013. A surprise 50th year anniversary party! Brilliant idea. We'll invite all of Mom and Lou's friends and family for a celebratory bash. Seeing all of his many cronies and colleagues would stimulate Lou and we'll have it at a local restaurant to make it easy to get to.

When we saw their car pull up we gave everybody the high sign. Fifty people stood in hushed expectation. When the door opened we all shouted, "Surprise!" The look on Mom's face was one of shock and delight. As her eyes swept the crowd her smile grew wider and brighter. Everybody she knew and loved was there. Then she saw, as did we all, the look on Lou's face. He recoiled in fear and confusion which quickly transformed to utter bewilderment. Mom guided him to a chair, explaining to everyone all the while, that he was happy they were all there and that he was just feeling tired.

It was a total disaster. From start to finish. Whatever level of cognition Lou had just then, in that moment, told him that everybody in the room now knew the depth of his disabilities even if he himself did not understand how compromised he was. First shame, then resentment flickered across his features and then he was gone, only the "befuddled Lou" remained. He couldn't or wouldn't interact with anyone at the party (we weren't sure which it was because sometimes when we looked at him he just appeared resentful and annoyed). Mom spent most of her time hovering over him, trying to act as an intermediary with all of the well-wishers.

We hadn't made anything better. We'd make it all so much worse.

*   *   *

From that day on, Lou's behavior became even more erratic. Any time he tried to walk, he stumbled. He couldn't control his arm movements. He was sleeping a lot and at odd times during the day. He would confuse the TV remote control with the lift-chair remote; unaware that the chair was lifting him to a semi-standing position, we would find him face down on the floor.

Then he would become perfectly coherent, but angry. He would lash out at Mom for putting his socks on him incorrectly. He yelled at Michael because something he wanted fixed (which wasn't actually broken) hadn't been handled.

"Let's talk," I said. *"You tell us Dad what is bothering you."* But he couldn't communicate what was wrong. The more he tried, the more he lost his train of thought, which made him jumble his words, which, (from our vantage point) made him appear short-tempered and impatient. We would try harder to encourage him to talk to us and he would try harder to respond, and the frustration carousel went round and round. He would glare at Mom because she, of all people, couldn't figure out what he was saying. Finally, he would give up and retreat into a sulky silence, obviously feeling sorry for himself.

So much had already been taken from this man; including his beloved Mercedes Benz. He knew what he wanted his body to do, but his brain was constantly misfiring so the tremors were randomly making his legs and arms jerk and spasm. He could no longer safely drive a car. The good news was that we got the keys away from him before he or anyone else was injured. The bad news was that every day for months Lou would look all around the house for his car keys. Each day he forgot he didn't have them and he would ask us where they were. Some days he got angry and demanded that we let him drive. Our refusal (regardless of accompanying explanations) was further proof that we were against him; that there was an enemy force occupying his home and we were it.

Perhaps at this point, you're wondering why my experience with Alzheimer's disease didn't automatically prepare me for what was going on. The fact is nobody was sure what was going on; Lou was not diagnosed with Alzheimer's and quite often he appeared perfectly aware even though he was incredibly moody and most always dissatisfied. Who wouldn't be given what was happening to his body? I understood that the Parkinson's disease decline would be progressive, his limbs were stiffening, his hands were like clubs so his fine motor skills were shot. However, I also learned that there is a world of difference between working at a residential facility to cognitively stimulate a non-combative resident vs. living inside a nightmare with an uncooperative, verbally and sometimes physically combative crazy person, twenty-four hours a day.

No job, no experience, no course, could have properly prepared me for the heart wrenching reality that was continuing to ramp up in intensity. Part of the reason I am writing this book, is to share that exact point. Even though I had education and experience, *nothing* could have taught me about what I was living. Except, perhaps, someone who had lived it before me.

*   *   *

Dawna Cappello and Susan Heller

Chapter 10
Medication and Madness

What if? What if we had understood the impact Lewy Body Dementia was having on Lou, from his perspective? Would we have refused to get him into a facility claiming we didn't want him drugged and turned into a zombie?

Susan Schneider Williams titled her article: "The Terrorist Inside My Husband's Brain", which turns out to be a horrifically accurate description of what we were seeing with Lou. Compounding our ignorance about the symptomology of his dementia were the conflicting side-effects of his numerous prescriptions. Apparently, many of the Parkinson's disease medications enhanced the dementia symptoms and many of the dementia medications exacerbated the Parkinson's disease symptoms.

Because we had Lou at home (meaning there was no on-site professional medical supervision), every time we introduced a new drug based on his latest symptoms, we had to wait a full two weeks to see if there was any positive response or adverse reaction. Based on that criteria, we had to stop whatever drug it was for another two weeks. Every single time. With every new prescription. Over seven years, including the early drug trials, the prescription count closes in on forty.

God only knows what impact the drug see-saw was having in Lou's already fractured world.

⌘
1.   Each disease causes symptoms that can magnify or mimic those of the other disease.
2.   Each medication can cause multiple side-effects.
3.   Each medication has side-effects that compound the negative drug interactions, or are completely contraindicated, meaning they could harm the patient or cause a life-threatening situation.

So one of the things I did during the final seven months, which would have been humongously helpful had I thought of it earlier, was to create two spreadsheets. One listed the side-effects possible for each medication and the other documented meds that were known in the medical literature to have negative interactions.

I used the computer program Excel, you can use stickies on a wall if you want to go low-tech. I included:

⌘
1.   The name of the drug.
2.   What it was supposed to address.
3.   The side-effects that were possible.
4.   The known interactions between drugs.
5.   The drugs that were definitely creating hideous reactions for Lou.

I'm not a doctor. The information below I gleaned from research on the Internet. This was just me trying to regain some control, some understanding of what this poor man was going through. The Parkinson's disease doctor is saying he has to take drugs A, B, and C, and the Lewy Body Dementia doc is saying, "Nah, Lou has to take drugs X, Y, and Z."

Here are samples from each of the spreadsheets I created. They may help you create a template for your specific situation.

⌘

The following medications can actually have up to 60 possible side-effects.

Sample Drug Symptoms & Side-Effects

MEDICATION:

GENERIC:	**Seroquel** (Quetiapine)
TAKEN FOR:	DEMENTIA
SYMPTOMS:	Memory & Psychosis
SIDE-EFFECTS:	Delusions, Depression, Confusion
GENERIC:	**Zoloft** (Sertraline)
TAKEN FOR:	PARKINSON'S
SYMPTOMS:	Anxiety
SIDE-EFFECTS:	Hallucinations, Hostility, Appetite
GENERIC:	**Carbidopa-Levodopa** (Sinemet)
TAKEN FOR:	PARKINSON'S
SYMPTOMS:	Shakiness, Stiff Body
SIDE-EFFECTS:	Vision Issues, Constipation, Anxiety

The following can actually have negative interactions with up to 300 disparate medications.

Sample Negative Prescription Interactions

MEDICATION:

GENERIC: **Seroquel** (Quetiapine)
TAKEN FOR: DEMENTIA
SYMPTOMS: Memory & Psychosis
INTERACTS WITH: Parkinson's Disease Medications, Anxiety Medications

GENERIC: **Zoloft** (Sertraline)
TAKEN FOR: PARKINSON'S
SYMPTOMS: Anxiety
INTERACTS WITH: Depression Medications, Anti-Inflammatory Medications

GENERIC: **Carbidopa-Levodopa** (Sinemet)
TAKEN FOR: PARKINSON'S
SYMPTOMS: Shakiness, Stiff Body
INTERACTS WITH: Dementia Medications, Blood Pressure Medications

It was agony watching Lou fight to stay present, fight to function as a father and a husband, and then have some drug that was supposed to help his blood pressure, or his memory, his prostate, his back pain, or his confusion, end up strapping him to a bucking demon of panic and impulsive behavior from which there seemed no escape. Which turned out to be true. There was no escape. This was only going in one direction. Had we known, had we understood, would we have been able to get past our own self-judgment, our own duty-bound insistence that we just put our heads into the wind and keep on keeping him at home?

None of us knew what the fight looked like from the inside of Lou's brain. We knew that the man was fighting, that's for damn sure. He made it clear that nothing was going to prevent him from doing his job as head of the family, as a man. When I learned the full reality of what his diagnosis did to people, almost a year after he died, it hit me like a ton of bricks. Though we experienced the outworking of the monsters through Lou's body, we never understood the depth of his suffering.

*   *   *

Chapter 11
It Gets Really Weird

One of the issues that started coming up was Lou's demand for sex. Voiced not just privately with Mom, but in front of Michael and me as well. He had lost his ability to function sexually a number of years earlier and Mom had given up trying with him. Seeking to protect his ego, she blamed the fact that they didn't have sex anymore on her recurring hip pain.

Now, Lou was adamant. He didn't remember that he was incapable so he would get upset and when that didn't work he tried manipulating her, saying things like, "What about my needs?" or "It's not fair to me." When Mom wouldn't acquiesce, Lou decided that meant she had to be sleeping with someone else.

If any man came into our home, regardless of his age, whether it was the computer guy, an electrician, a neighbor, or even any of our male family members, Lou was convinced that they were having an affair with Mom. He knew she was cheating because he was sure he saw men coming in and out of the house during all hours of the day and night. His extreme jealousy and mistrust grew. Any time the phone rang, he would pick up the extension next to his chair and listen in. He was certain it was a man calling for Mom.

Although Michael and I worked as a team with Mom on a daily basis, we had also begun to make sure that she got a full day out of the house once in a while. Her favorite thing was to go to the casino and play Bingo. Unfortunately, any degree of relief or respite was instantly wiped out by Lou's accusations and his demand for sex as soon as she walked in the door to prove she wasn't cheating. She ended up expending so much energy defending herself and answering his probing questions that she would end up more drained than before she left. It was too high a price to pay. She stopped going. We could see she was reaching the end of her rope.

Then, Lou became positively obsessed about asking for sex. It turned into an all-consuming issue, so much so that he told Mom he would rather die than not have sex anymore and if he did die, it would be her fault. Mom was crushed. Michael decided he had to step in and have a man-to-man conversation with his father. The difficulty we now realize, was that Lou truly couldn't process what was being said. The facts and words were not connecting with his brain. At the time, his gruff and surly attitude made it appear that he was simply refusing to have the discussion and he waved Michael away.

I couldn't think of what else to do so I decided to write messages on note-cards and placed them in and around Lou's environment, as sort of silent feedback reminders. *"Lou and Barb do not have sex anymore, and it's ok. They show their love with hugs."* Michael made sure that every time Mom went out to do errands, just before she returned, he would remind his father not to ask his mother for sex, but to just reach out and hug her. The whole thing was fraught with embarrassment and incredibly uncomfortable for us, but it was the only thing we could think of to do.

Surprisingly, the notecards seemed to help, so we began expanding them to include everything that was happening that day and made sure to hang them in specific locations throughout the house.

⌘

Things like:

1.　　The day of the week.
2.　　The specific month.
3.　　The current season.
4.　　The activities of the day.

If Mom was heading out we created cards that said:

1.　　What time she was going out.
2.　　Where she was going.
3.　　Who she was going to be with.
4.　　What time she would be home.

　　　The intensity and frequency of Lou's requests for sex diminished but he refocused his anxiety and agitation on the other potent trigger for blow-ups, money. He knew beyond a shadow of a doubt that we were spending all of the money he had invested for the future, demanding to be shown checkbook registers and online investments. The fuel for that fire was, of course, that he could no longer reconcile which numbers meant what and he most definitely did not want to hear any lies about the costs of medication, doctors, and tests. He was on to us, we had altered everything, it was all just one ongoing betrayal.

　　　　　*　　　　　*　　　　　*

Chapter 12
Technology Rules

As Lou's mind continued to deteriorate he began wandering inside of the house, often heading toward one of the doors that led outside. Constant vigilance was required. One day, Mom dared to take a shower while Lou was napping in his chair. She came out to find his chair empty. She ran through the house calling him. She looked in all the bedrooms, taking time to double check the closets. No Lou.

She flew upstairs calling his name, over and over. No response. Finally, she headed for the basement. Around every corner, down every flight of stairs, her heart skipped a beat, terrified by what she might find. "Please, please, please, please, please," was the refrain in her brain. Lou had disappeared.

When she finally found him, he was outside, almost naked, sitting in his car.

That's when we realized we needed to avail ourselves of some very simple technology.

⌘

1.   We bought motion sensors and video cameras.
2.   We used baby monitors in every room.
3.   We utilized intercoms for instant communication.

The motion sensors were installed in every doorway so we could track Lou's movements in the house. As difficult as it could be for him to move his body, he certainly seemed to be able to fight his way to a standing position and get out of his chair at the most inopportune times. Was he as compromised as we thought or was he being cagey? We couldn't figure it out and none of his doctors had the answer either.

Sometimes, Lou would be almost sweet, although he never smiled. His energy could be soft and it was clear he was doing his best to cooperate with us. Once, after Lou sneezed, Michael said to his father, "God Bless You" and Lou said, "He already did. He gave me you." Another time, Mom was reciting a list of all the people who loved and cared for Lou, and before she could finish mentioning the names she hoped he would remember, he called out, "Don't forget my daughter-in-law." Those moments were the exception and they were becoming fewer and fewer. Some days he would be continuously combative and difficult.

The Deadly Duo (as I have come to think of them) of Parkinson's disease and Lewy Body dementia, combined to reduce Lou's mobility by making his body rigid. Mom could barely escort him through the house on her own anymore. He would lean on her arm and shoulder not realizing how heavy he was, seeking the balance he needed in order to walk. However, because Lou was barely able to lift his feet from the floor, the long, arduous process of shuffling across the carpet was hugely taxing on both of them.

Getting dressed was also an ordeal. Once Mom finally succeeded in wrestling Lou to wherever he needed to be, she would then have to get him into a sitting position. Next, she had to summon all her strength to literally lift his arms in order to get his upper body into a shirt. She would have to pause to catch her breath, and then, after raising each leg for him, she would shimmy them into his pants and finally get him standing again so she could pull them up and they could begin the long, slow trip back across the floor.

⌘

A range of adaptive clothing for people with limited mobility is now available. I'm not connected in any way to the following companies, I found them on the Internet.

1.   www.buckandbuck.com
2.   www.silverts.com/shop-by-need

One night, Mom said she was feeling dizzy. Her chest felt heavy and she began having heart palpitations. Lou was extremely worried. He struggled to get out of his chair to get her to the Emergency Room. Michael had already gone for the car.

Mom was looking at Dad, fear clearly written across her face. But before he could reach her, his brain pulled the reality-rug out from under him. As Michael bundled Mom into the car, Lou was left standing in extreme confusion, unable to make sense of what was going on around him.

*   *   *

Chapter 13
Plan B. And C...and D.

Time for a new plan. The ER doc said Mom's blood pressure was through the roof, so now she too, was on medication. Mom and Lou had been givers and doers all their lives, neither one of them had a frame of reference for asking for help outside the family. However, she now understood that she needed more support, so I pushed my agenda for having her attend a support group for caregivers dealing with dementia.

That meant there was another line we would have to cross with Lou because Mom would be leaving the house more often. So be it, because if Michael and I were feeling fried, she was beyond pan seared and burned.

It worked. Mom saw and heard her story mirrored in many different ways, from all kinds of different people.

⌘

1. AARP
   Online, (or through your local library) is a tremendous resource.
2. ALZHEIMER'S RESOURCE CENTERS
   In all 50 states, (check online or through your local library) offer knowledge, support, and resources to care for loved ones with dementia.
3. HELPGUIDE.ORG
   Is an organization that collaborates with Harvard University, and has a comprehensive online presentation that specifically addresses Lewy Body Dementia.
4. NAMI (National Alliance on Mental Illness)
   Is a grassroots organization, focused on providing support and information as well as advocating for public policy.

One of the roughest duties Mom had to contend with was Lou's hygiene. She found it easy enough to fill his toothbrush with toothpaste and to brush his hair for him every morning. However, Lou's body was so very unstable;

trying to maneuver him in the shower, keep him from falling, and wash him with a bar of soap, was back-breaking work for a woman who was also in her 70's.

We decided that Michael would take over Lou's personal hygiene routine. Moving forward, he was going to be the one to shower and dress his father every morning before he left for work, or if Lou happened to be too tired on any given morning, Michael would take care of those tasks as soon as he got home.

You see what I mean about Michael? Not many men would be willing to undertake such a difficult and emotionally charged task. It was hard work, Lou clearly was not happy and it certainly wasn't something Michael relished doing. But Michael is a Cappello; when somebody is in need, they show up and get the job done.

Next up, was a plan to increase Lou's confidence in himself. I designed a series of exercises that would help stimulate his mind and keep his body moving.

This is where my work at the Alzheimer's Resource Center did come into play.

⌘

I learned how to engage six of the brain's cognitive domains:
1. Reaction Time
2. Language
3. Visual-Spatial
4. Attention & Concentration
5. Memory
6. Problem Solving

I showed him pictures and prompted him with basic questions about boating and travel to the places he had once loved. At first, his eyes lit up when he saw familiar photographs and he seemed eager to play along. Then his brain would misfire, he couldn't find the words he wanted, and he would immediately shut down. Though I consistently redirected him, and at times was able to guide his attention back on task, as soon as he realized he wasn't performing well, he stopped trying.

So how could we say Lou wasn't "present" when he knew enough to know that his memory was letting him down? When he was cognizant enough to be discomfited to the point of acute embarrassment by his inability to name the connections with people and places he had once treasured.

My next attempt was to try physical exercises that I thought he would find entertaining and might even keep him motivated. I got out my hand-held punching pad and a pair of boxing gloves. Just putting the gloves on Lou proved to be a lengthy form of physical therapy (for both of us) but once they were on, the look on his face and his effort to sit up straight told me that I'd finally hit pay dirt.

I began by standing in front of him while he was sitting in his chair, holding the punching pad at a good level for him. *"Punch one time with your right hand, Slugger."* And he did. *"Now the left hand, punch hard!"* He got that too. So I slowly increased the number of punches per hand. If nothing else, I was hoping to tire him out in a positive way.

And here we revisit some of the crazy-making stuff for caregivers dealing with any level of dementia. Although he was often confused about so many other things, just as with the photographs, Lou quickly became aware that he wasn't doing well. He had a hard time lifting his arms, his swings were awkward and lacked control. When he managed to land a punch it barely connected. Despite my encouragement, he refused to continue, he very clearly knew he wasn't doing it "right" and it upset him. He was ashamed and embarrassed. Which brings us right back to our confusion about his confusion. What does he know? When does he know it? Is he truly crazy, or was our collective exhaustion and frustration making us the crazy ones?

*   *   *

Chapter 14
Denial. Definitely Not a River in Egypt.

Mom, Michael, and I had no personal lives. We left the house to go to work, buy groceries, and go to doctor's appointments. Taking care of Lou took all three of us doing what we came to consider "our heart-work". It had been almost a decade, during which time we gradually learned to stop taking any negative responses or misdirected actions personally. That said, it was getting increasingly difficult to manage him, though there was one moment in time when we thought we had figured out what was really going on.

Michael was on Lou-watch and saw him grab a pill that was on the bathroom sink and pop it in his mouth. It could have been a spot of toothpaste, a drop of hand cream, or a tiny piece of tissue paper, Lou couldn't tell the difference. The very next day, Mom saw him grab a handful of pills and before she could stop him they were down the hatch. Aha! we thought. That's it. Lou has been overmedicating, taking who knows what combination of pharmaceuticals. So we're not completely nuts, he is in there, it's just that he's been zonked out on random combinations of pills.

All of this made a weird kind of sense because there were some through-lines that Lou held onto until the bitter end. The sex thing still came up as did his suspicions that we were taking him to the financial cleaners. There was the almost-always successful lure of chocolate-raspberry ice cream, and finally, what we took to calling Lou's pill-crazy-sanity. Because, even if he didn't recall one single memory in a day, he always remembered that he had to take his pills. Which brings up yet another hugely troubling question for the truth search-engine that is hindsight; was he seeking the equivalent of the mental "drug holiday" that is given to people in nursing homes whose brains are delivering non-stop nightmares, dread, and violent hallucinations?

Once Lou passed out after taking the additional pills, Michael and I gathered all of his medications and hid them in a closet in our apartment. Believing that we finally had a reasonable explanation for all the weird behavior variations, Mom, Michael, and I experienced a profound sense of relief even though we knew he was going to be mad as hell when he couldn't find them.

We were right. And we were wrong. We were right because Lou was beyond furious when he couldn't find his pills, he was livid. He knew (and this time he was right) that we had conspired to remove them; another betrayal. He shut down entirely, refusing to speak to us or acknowledge our existence for days. Mom was devastated; she couldn't stop crying and decided we had to give him back his medications. Michael and I refused, which made us feel terrible because now both she and Lou were in deep states of despair.

Over the following week, we watched anxiously for the positive changes we anticipated in Lou's behavior since we were now in charge of his meds. This would be where we were wrong. There weren't any. He was constantly dizzy, falling asleep, and his mood swings were abrupt and precipitous. In the course of a single hour he could process through five different presentations; from fairly calm to downright nasty, and everything in-between. He was living the most wretched life, trapped inside himself in ways we didn't begin to understand.

Perhaps due to my background and the fact that, as a daughter-in-law, I was one-step removed from the drama, I had a slightly broader perspective than my husband and Mom. When I worked at the Alzheimer's Resource Center I had heard people discussing virtual reality simulations for caregivers of Parkinson's disease patients, so I checked it out, and because I had to stay home with Lou, I set up a tour for Mom and Michael. I thought it would deepen their understanding of what Lou was up against and help them identify with what it was like to be inside his head and body.

That was my denial because I didn't realize that they absolutely could not accept (nor could I) that the man we loved was suffering so horrifically, and still honor our promise not to put him in a nursing home. So they turned the experience into a game. The exercises were designed to provide insight into Lou's mind; how it was filled with annoying chatter and endless commotion, and to illustrate how distorted and disorienting the visual and auditory information he was receiving could be.

⌘

The Virtual Reality Tour was comprised of three devices worn at the same time:

1. Headphones that continuously delivered disruptive sounds like beeping, hissing, static, and weird echoing noises.
2. Goggles that randomly shifted between tunnel vision and moving bright lights, which could trigger full-body motion sickness.
3. Big, clunky, oversized gloves that made it almost impossible to lift and maneuver anything.

While wearing all of the items above, Michael and Mom were asked to focus on and identify specific words that were being recited to them while counting how many items were placed in front of them. They accepted the challenge and even competed to see who would score better, but they were both astonished by how many times they got it wrong.

They were literally hearing through Lou's ears and seeing through Lou's eyes.

In addition, they were given everyday tasks to accomplish while keeping all three of the gadgets on: folding clothes, setting a table, and filling up a glass of water. Even though they had expected to be able to accomplish the simple assignments successfully, they quickly found out how much effort was required to even attempt them. In the end, the folded clothes were all over the place, the table was a mess, and the water was not so much in the glass as splashed on the counter all around the glass.

The tour was supposed to help them understand all that Lou was experiencing on a daily basis. The cold hard truth was, based on the need to survive *their* current reality, they came away joking about the whole experience. They could not begin to extrapolate what had happened to them with what was going on inside of Lou. **

*   *   *

** The same peer-reviewed authority, The Official Journal of the American Academy of Neurology, that published Susan Schneider Williams' article about her husband, also published an article about the difficulty and confusion in the medical community diagnosing Parkinson's disease psychosis (PDP). Published April 16, 2016 - **Experiencing Parkinson's Disease Psychosis via Virtual Reality Simulation: A Novel and Effective Educational Tool** (P1.011). You can read the article abstract here: www.neurology.org/content/86/16_Supplement/P1.011.

Chapter 15
Signs & Portents

Due to the degree of Lou's impairment, Michael wanted the baby monitors that we had set up in our bedroom upstairs over a year earlier, to be on twenty-four hours a day. Lou's night-terror hallucinations were ramping up. We would finally have fallen asleep after an exhausting day when suddenly, Lou would cry out. Flying down to his room we would find him standing in a guarded position, dangerously teetering, as he held an imaginary gun pointed at an empty corner of the room; his face white as a ghost, with a look of horror that could not be mistaken for anything but a genuine fear for his life.

Sometimes, we'd find him lying in his bed whimpering, covers clutched up to his chin, frantically pointing with one hand at some fearsome something that was menacing him. First we tried reassuring him, walking around the room waving our arms to show him nothing and nobody was there. It didn't work. Then we tried engaging with the monsters, ordering them out of the room, mock fighting and killing them. That didn't work either. Because, as we now understand, the evil monsters were very much in residence, they were 100% real and we were the ones who couldn't see them.

If the monsters held sway through the night, in the morning we would be faced with an exhausted, miserable, and combative man, one we still couldn't reach because all he could see and hear were the terrorists pursuing him. Some mornings he could recall the nighttime battlefield and would accuse us of conspiring with the "people of the night" to harm and abduct him.

If he wasn't "hallucinating", he was repeatedly calling Mom even if he didn't need anything. Because of Lou's uncontrollable body tremors, Mom would be kept awake by the shaking of his arm against her back or the quaking of the bed, so she hadn't slept with him for years. That meant she had to get up and go into his room. When she did, he would say, "Hi." He didn't want water or need to go to the bathroom; he was lonely and just wanted company. But by 10:00 at night, Mom was exhausted and desperately needed downtime.

Lou's pleas for attention pulled on all of our heartstrings, the whole situation was just so indescribably sad. Michael and I took over night-time duty, which could mean getting up between eight and fifteen times a night, sometimes more. Lou never slept through the night.

However, this meant that he was truly the only one in the household getting any attention. Mom was never center stage. We wanted to make sure they both received attention as well as positive reinforcement. Lou was still stoically (unknowingly?) refusing to express any appreciation for everything Mom did during the day, so Michael and I began a propaganda campaign. *"Thank you!"* we would call out loudly to her every time she did something for us, or for him. We were saying the words "Thank you" over fifty times a day in Lou's presence, hoping it would rub off on him, even a little bit.

We continued our vocal "Thank you" efforts for several weeks, when finally, out of the blue, Lou began saying "Thank you" once in a while. If Michael was around and his mother did something for his father, Michael would encourage him to thank her. Even though Lou may not have been able to remember on his own, he would say the words and the effect on Mom was immediate. She lit up; it was the only sign of love she had received from her husband in years.

One day I went downstairs to check in, as I did every morning. Lou was sitting in his living room chair, his eyes unfocused but staring in my direction. I loudly and cheerfully said, *"Good morning Dad!"* His eyes popped open wide as he pulled focus and joyfully replied, "Thank you!" We laughed about that for days.

So you see, you can sometimes make inroads and other times touch hearts. Lou's response was a reminder that though he was not able to show us the kind and gentle man that we all knew him to have been, his loving spirit was still somewhere inside of his ailing body and mind.

Another effort we made was to say, "I love you" to Mom in front of Lou, hoping it would prompt him to say it to her. Whether it was in the morning when we first saw each other or before going to bed, or even after she did something nice for us, it was our way of telling her how much we loved and appreciated her.

In addition, we went public with one small gesture that Michael and I had shared during our life together. Whenever the clock showed any repeating number like, 10:10a.m. or 3:33p.m., I would holler, *"Love you"* so no matter where Michael was in the house he could hear me. We began doing the same thing when we were downstairs with Mom and Lou, we would even open the door at the top of the stairs and yell down, *"Love you"* to them at those specific times.

One morning we were sitting together in their downstairs living room watching television. Lou startled all three of us by bellowing, "Love you!" at the top of his lungs. We looked at him and then at each other, delightfully surprised. Then Mom pointed to the clock. It was 11:11a.m.

*　　　　　*　　　　　*

Dawna Cappello and Susan Heller

Chapter 16
Call in The Cavalry

One night we just snapped. Michael, Mom, and I. It wasn't pretty and we aren't proud of it, but clearly we had been heading toward this place for a long time.

Tension had been building for months. During the day Lou was prowling the house having fought us and his own body to get out of his chair each and every time. Protecting the family was Lou's job and nothing was going to stop him. He would go to the windows, fearful of what he would find. The men with guns that were waiting to kill us all. The guy who was secretly planting a bomb in Mom's car.

Suddenly, the monster in his brain would yank a lever, the slot machine tumblers would spin, and bing, bang, bong, there they were; three skull & crossbones. So then, when he would get to the windows, he'd start punching the glass, screaming that we were keeping him in jail; desperate to get somebody's attention, he was begging for someone to rescue *him*.

It was one of those nights when we couldn't get Lou to go to bed, never mind sleep. He resisted going into his room, he was being really nasty to Mom and querulous with us. The three of us were bone-tired and wanted nothing more than to go to bed ourselves. It was not to be. After hours of negotiating, bribing, arguing, and pleading, we finally got him into bed.

I remember trudging up the stairs my legs feeling like lead, I think I brushed my teeth though I may have simply assumed that. The next thing I knew, Michael and I were racing downstairs. I don't remember getting into bed or falling asleep, but in fact, only half an hour had passed when Lou started to scream. We were all the way down the stairs before my brain caught up with what my body was doing.

Lou was seeing things, pointing in all different directions, which had Mom, Michael, and I darting around the room, banging into each other. Lou became enraged because our frantic movements were making whatever he was seeing, worse. Suddenly, we were all screaming at each other, screaming at Lou, demanding to know why he didn't believe us. *"There's nothing there Dad,"* I screeched over and over, *"There's nothing there!"*

Michael was yelling at Lou to stop yelling, Mom was hysterical. At one point during the chaos Lou shouted, "I don't know, I'm all over the place!" with a look of such pure anguish on his face, we all burst into tears.

Finally, after we'd cried it out and calmed down, we got Lou back to bed. He was wiped out. *"This has to stop, it has to change,"* I said in a whisper, my voice hoarse from screaming. *"We're shouting at each other like reckless idiots, we're shouting at him, we're not doing this right, we're not doing a good job anymore."* And then I pointed out that the three of us were living for the one who was slowly dying, and that was draining the very life out of us as well.

What I didn't realize at the time, what none of us understood, was that the only way Lou could be spared his downward spiraling nightmare was through sedation. The other thing we hadn't considered but you may want to if you are anywhere along this illness continuum, is adult daycare; something that would have been appropriate for Lou at least six of the seven years when he was really suffering.

Mom and Michael felt that they had to honor their promise to Lou to keep him home, but what I've learned since he died, was that we weren't doing him any favors. Like a child who has to have a shot, you need to know there will be upset and then it will pass. Lou would likely have kicked up a fuss initially, then he would have been entirely engaged with the activities and the professional caregivers.

Dawna Cappello and Susan Heller

Lou needed stimulation and engagement, not just babysitting; we didn't realize that boredom meant the monsters would have free rein.

Inadvertently, we were also risking his life. More than a dozen times when Michael and I were both at work, Lou had hit the deck. Mom wasn't strong enough to get him back to his feet. She'd get a pillow and blanket and wait next to him until Michael or I were able to get home. The first time it happened she called 911. Big mistake, and as far as she was concerned, one she would never make again unless she saw broken bones or blood flowing. The hospital kept him strapped to a hard plastic gurney for six hours. The man was terrified, his back was in agony, and the bloody monsters parlayed the misery of his entrapment in every torqued and twisted way imaginable.

So we did our best, Michael still took him out on the boat even when Lou required a wheelchair, but just letting him be at home, sitting in front of the TV, and bribing him with ice-cream, was nowhere near enough input for the man. Adult daycare offers cognitive challenges, games that help mobility, specially designed exercises, socialization, and connection with loving professionals, any one of whom could have rescued Lou from the floor. Most facilities can dispense medications and importantly, protocols and strategies in case of emergencies are part of any reputable program.

Additionally, and here's the part that breaks my heart to admit, they could have helped us understand when Lou crossed the line and assisted us in getting him into a facility where appropriate sedation could have spared him some of the hideous trauma that was free-ranging in his brain. The difference in the quality of life that would have made for him and for us is beyond description. We didn't know, but now, you do. Here are some resources from the Internet to check out.

⌘

Adult Daycare Resources for Lewy Body Dementia, Parkinson's and Alzheimer's diseases:

1. LEWY BODY DEMENTIA
   www.lbda.org/content/new-study-shows-caregivers-benefit-adult-day-services
2. PARKINSON'S DISEASE
   www.agingcare.com/parkinsons-disease
3. ALZHEIMER'S DISEASE
   www.alz.org/care/alzheimers-dementia-adult-day- centers.asp
4. ALZHEIMER'S RESOURCE CENTER OF CT, INC.
   www.arc-ct.org/adult_day_programs.php

*   *   *

Chapter 17

Just So You Know.

This is How it Played Out for Lou.

You know Lou well enough by now to imagine how the idea of strangers in the house was going to set him off, but we absolutely had no choice. We were out of our league and we finally had to admit it. It was very difficult for Mom and Michael to discuss what was happening to Lou, they would both become so emotional they couldn't really hear what was being said, so I became the voice of the family. I called Lou's neurologist for a recommendation for in-home support.

And it gets really weird. Again.

Lou was perfectly *fine* about a nurse coming into our house, in fact, he was kind of amazing. As soon as she walked in the door his symptoms damn near disappeared! How was that even possible? He wasn't leaning as far forward while walking, he was sitting up straighter in his chair, and he was speaking more clearly than he had in weeks.

Then it hit us. Lou was trying to impress her. He had a plan in place. Seriously? He was going to prove that he was fine and that we were being alarmist, or worse. Maybe we were resentful family members who didn't want to be bothered taking care of him. Clearly, he needed to be the one in charge of his own medication, we were not to be trusted.

Collectively, we were dumbstruck. Mom was heartbroken. If he could rally like this for a complete stranger, what did that say about his feelings for her? For us?

We had to keep reminding ourselves that what was left of Lou's mind had gone back in time, it was like he was a child again; getting what he wanted, how he wanted it, and when he wanted it. It had nothing to do with us and what we did or didn't do for him.

However, it quickly became clear Lou realized he wasn't going to convince anyone that he could control his own medication. He began fighting the physical therapists the nurse had scheduled for him, he was alternately afraid of the aides we'd finally hired to help us out, and then trying to protect them. From us.

It started when Michael found Lou gouging out huge handfuls of goopy lotion in the bathroom. As he tried to steer his father's hands toward the sink Lou went ballistic. Michael couldn't get a grip on him because his hands were unbelievably slippery. It turned into a full-on altercation. Desperately trying to prevent his father from falling, Michael took repeated punches to his face until he could get Lou stabilized, then he just backed away. Michael's left eye was bleeding, his right cheek was swollen, and his clothes were torn. It was harrowing.

That same night when the home health aide arrived for her shift, Lou, who could barely shuffle his feet, actually ran to her. Grabbing her arm, he pointed to Michael and me screaming, "These are the killers, and *we* are the killees!" Then he rushed her to the back bedroom slamming the door shut to keep her safe.

Our bodies are comprised of two systems; chemical and electrical. Lou's fight or flight system temporarily overrode the monsters that had invaded his brain and body. Even though we wanted to believe it meant Lou was still there, he wasn't. He hadn't been for a long time.

Now, any time one of us came within arm's length of him, he would grab, hit, or growl at us (or a combination of all three). When he did succeed in getting hold of us, his grip was incredibly strong, fear and adrenaline providing him power we'd no idea he still possessed. He would twist our fingers or wrists and absolutely would not let go. The real Lou Cappello would never, ever, have hurt a soul. Even we had to admit the man we knew was no longer present.

Suddenly, Lou stopped sleeping, eating, and going to the bathroom. He couldn't walk, couldn't sit down, couldn't lie down, he couldn't speak and when he tried, what came out were moans and guttural cries.

It had long ago been agreed that I would be the one to make the decision when the time came; Mom and Michael were not capable of making the call.

Though Mom was completely hysterical, she knew, we no longer had a choice. Crying, I turned to Michael and said, *"Honey, I'm making the call."* Michael looked straight at me, expressionless. I watched as the blood drained from his face, he was the starkest shade of white. Then, his features scrunched up so tightly I barely recognized him. He sank to his knees heartsick and sobbing, his tears flowing like I had never seen in my entire life. I stood in shock and watched my husband break into a million pieces.

Hands shaking I reached for my phone, trying to get the words out around the sobs that were choking me. *"What can we do to get our Dad into your facility today? We will pay cash. He needs your help so terribly."*

Lou only lived eight more days. He was almost comatose at first, then he became violent. The physical outbursts alternated with fits of sobbing, which ripped our hearts apart. The doctor asked, "What facility did Lou come to us from?" When we told her we had brought him straight from home, she, the nurses, and staff were flabbergasted-- they just couldn't believe it. Lou was so overpoweringly aggressive he was increased to a four person assist. He also became a danger to the other patients. Finally, the doctors helped us understand that he could stay where he was in the deepest and darkest of hells, or we could move him to a facility where he could receive the "drug holiday". That lasted three days, and then Lou was gone. The date was April 21, 2016.

*　　　　　*　　　　　*

Chapter 18
You Gotta Let the Guilt Go...

Here's why. In some ways, the guilt piece can actually be a selfish thing. Not intentionally or even consciously, but I can look back and see how many times Mom, Michael, and I reassured one another and ourselves that we were doing the right thing for Lou. It made us feel better, stronger, maybe even special.

Family and friends were shocked to hear how quickly Lou's condition had deteriorated once he arrived at the nursing facility, but that was our fault. We knew that their disbelief was because we had kept all of the atrocious experiences, the drama, and the ongoing trauma to ourselves, thinking we were protecting Lou. We weren't, and had we talked openly about what was going on, we likely would have been informed by someone, somewhere, that there were options that would have been better for everybody.

The truth is, if Lou had been in adult daycare it would have allowed us to interact *with* him as opposed to just reacting *to* him. Would it have made a difference to him? That's impossible to answer though I fully believe the answer is yes. Helping hearts and hands feel energetically different when they're proffered through a haze of exhaustion, fear, frustration, and yes, sometimes resentment. How much more patient and joyous might we have been with him if we weren't on-call twenty-four hours a day? We'll never know. Would adult daycare have slowed down the progression of the monsters? Probably not. Could it have helped him feel more connected to the world around him? Nobody knows the answer to that question. Yet.

Which brings us full circle back to Susan Schneider Williams' article addressed to doctors and researchers. She wrote: "I know you have accomplished much already in the areas of research and discovery toward cures in brain disease. And I am sure at times the progress has felt painfully slow. Do not give up. Trust that a cascade of cures and discovery is imminent in all areas of brain disease and you will be a part of making that happen."

Mom, Michael, and I second her belief and faith that science will find a way to address the terrorists of the brain. Meanwhile, if you're a caregiver, take heart, take care of yourselves, and share what it is that you've learned, what you know. Somebody, somewhere needs to hear that they're not alone in the drama.

⌘

1. LBDU - LEWY BODY DEMENTIA UNIVERSITY
   www.lbda.org/node/4 - (Community Forum)
2. DEMENTIA CAREGIVER SUPPORT - ONLINE
   www.dementiacarecentral.com/caregiverinfo/online-support/
3. PARKINSON'S DISEASE - DEMENTIA FORUM
   www.dementiaforum.org/learn-more/diseases/parkinsons-disease/
4. ALZHEIMER'S ASSOCIATION
   www.alzconnected.org

Afterword

Following Lou's death there was a huge outpouring of love. Hundreds of friends, family, employees, and colleagues from all over the country came to the services; a true testament to the exquisite man who had been Lou Cappello.

After the wake, we received a tiny stained glass lamp that stays lit at all times to signify Lou's presence of light still shining in our lives. Every time Michael and I walk by the lamp we say, *"Hi Dad"*, as a way of keeping him alive in our hearts.

Finally, after the cremation, we put his ashes in a biodegradable sea shell and drove up to what had been his beloved marina. Together we placed the shell into the ocean and watched Lou's spirit float away to freedom.

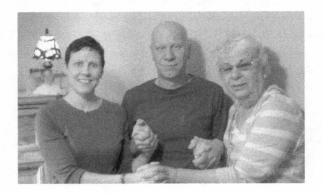

Epilogue
Mike & Mom

MICHAEL CAPPELLO

"Only eight days. I kept my father home for all of his life, except for eight days." That's what I said to Dawna as we walked out after Dad died. I was crying my eyes out, but I felt like I'd done right by him.

It's been a year and some, and I've learned a lot about the bastards who took over my father's world. Here's what I can tell you I've learned about the diseases; sometimes it's luck and sometimes genetics. In my family the genetic thing is big. I've written into my will specifics about what I do and don't want done if the monsters come for me. No suffering. No need to pretend I'm "in there" when I'm not. Do what you gotta do and go for the drug holiday the second I've crossed the line.

I don't want anyone to go through what Dad, Mom, Dawna, and I did. Whoever you are, I hope this helps.

MOM (BARBARA CAPPELLO)

Over half a century together. How do you say goodbye? I couldn't. So maybe if I'd understood the torture Lou was going through in his head, if someone could've explained there were OK choices, it might have been different. I can't judge what we did and didn't do, all I know is, it's what we did. I'm glad that Dawna found a way for you to know about the options. Like Mike said, I don't want anybody else to suffer because they didn't know.

And whoever you are, I'm praying for you.

This book is dedicated to my husband Michael.

Thank you for all of the ways you support me.

Thank you for sharing your loving parents with me.

Being your wife is one of my greatest blessings.

To my mother-in-law Barbara:

Thank you for being my Mom.

It is a privilege to be your daughter.